Conquering
the *Beast* Within

Conquering
the *Beast* Within

How I Fought Depression and Won . . .

and How You Can, Too

Written and Illustrated by

Cait Irwin

Previously titled *Depression: Challenge the Beast Within Yourself . . . and Win*

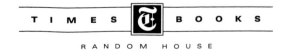

TIMES BOOKS

RANDOM HOUSE

YA
616.85
IRWIN

This book is Cait Irwin's personal account of her battle with depression. It is in no way meant to take the place of expert advice from a health care professional. It is sold with the understanding that neither the author nor the publisher are engaged in rendering professional advice.

CONTENTS

Acknowledgments

Deep love and special thanks to my family, especially my mother who has been with me through my whole ordeal. Thanks to my Grandma Sue, her friends and Aunt Sis for all their prayer chains ranging from Council Bluffs to Ireland!!!!! All my cousins, aunts, uncles and friends of our family have given me so much support. Our sweet pets, Huey, Tex and Glynis gave me so much comfort. Thanks to the St. Albert High School staff for getting me through a terribly tough school year, especially to Ms. McGuire and Ms. Mooney who are the most loving teachers. Good friends are hard to come by. Thanks, Michala, Mandy, Ellen, Liz, Jill, Val, Sharon, the Colemans, Annie Bendalin, Ione Jenson for all your love and encouragement.

Thanks Dr. Michael Meyer, for being the best psychiatrist in Omaha. Thank you, Susan Carter-Rothe, for being the best therapist in Omaha.

Last, but not least, I want to thank my business "Pard" whose patience and perseverance has made this book possible. I love you, Uncle Spark!

Preface

Depression is widespread. Studies indicate that nearly a third of all of the families in the country have had one or more of their family members suffer from a bout with severe depression. Also affecting families is the fact that depression-related suicide is a leading cause of death in young people age 15 to 24.

According to the American Psychiatric Association, "one of the biggest problems is that people do not understand depression and even deny its existence."

In her book, *Conquering the Beast Within*, Cait Irwin has created a powerful visual image of depression that adolescents and adults can relate to, and even children can understand. It graphically examines the feelings and emotions of depression, explains how depression affects the individual as well as family members and friends, and details the necessary steps to recovery.

By creating this personal metaphor, Cait was able to understand and deal with her own depression. At 13, Cait began struggling with depression, feeling it as a consuming sadness growing into a beast that gobbled up her self-esteem, confidence, trust, and love of life. Like many other teenagers, Cait was at a point where she could no longer cope and considered suicide. Fortunately she told her mother and was hospitalized. As part of her recovery process Cait began to accurately chronicle her depression and the suggested techniques for dealing with this illness in a creative, visual journal. Out of her sincere desire to help others, Cait has refined her images, thoughts, feelings, techniques, and experiences and made it available for the benefit of all who are in any way connected with depression.

This book is dedicated to anyone who has been touched in some way by depression. Breaking out and regaining one's freedom, with a lighthearted feeling, is what this book is all about. It is also in memory of the people whose lives were taken by depression.

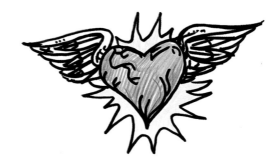

Conquering
the *Beast* Within

CHAPTER ONE

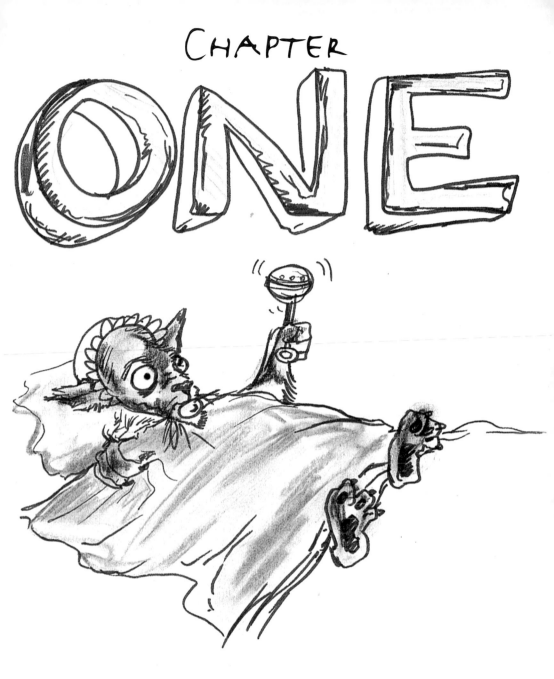

A BEAST IS BORN

In our minds stalks a beast... a cruel, mean and wicked beast. This beast loves to hate. He is that feeling you have when you say, "I give up", or "I hate myself" or "I don't want to live". He loves to devour your good feelings.

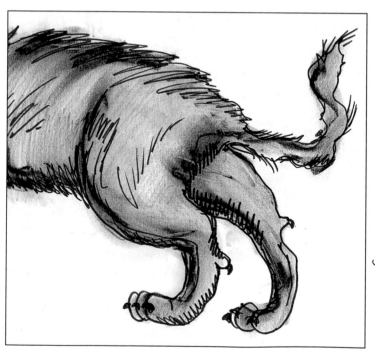

He eats everything that matters to you til you are left with nothing...

The Beast is Depression!

During my personal struggle with depression I began to see a wild and ferocious beast as a symbol of my illness. Seeing the beast as a separate being helped me to understand and cope with the way I was feeling. Hopefully, my perspective of the beast will help you and those around you understand the illness, its emotions,

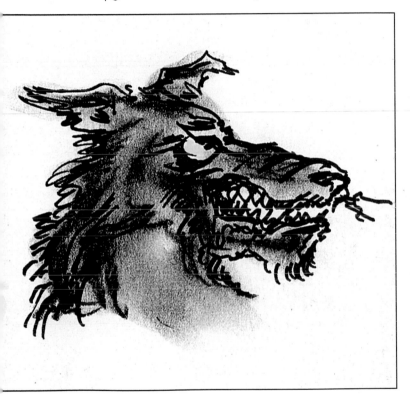

reactions, and feelings, which may be hard to explain. I had to make a decision to either challenge the beast or give in to him. Sometimes you might think it's easier just to give up and live with depression, or give up and let go of life. I decided to challenge him everyday until I won. You have the courage and persistence in your heart to challenge your beast and be a winner.

Some people refer to depression as a mental illness or brain disorder. I call it my broken leg theory. Let me explain. While I was depressed I missed a lot of things; the many great times I could have had with my friends and family; a bunch of school; and my favorite sports. I basically felt like I had missed a huge portion of my life. I felt terrible but my family and friends helped me to realize that what I have is an illness, just like having a broken leg. If you broke your leg you would miss out on some school and sports and other activities. You'd still have to do a lot of work to get better. If you had a serious disease like cancer you would have to do a lot of work to feel better, like taking medicine and enduring pain, (physical and mental). Just remember your depression, the beast, is just as serious and real.

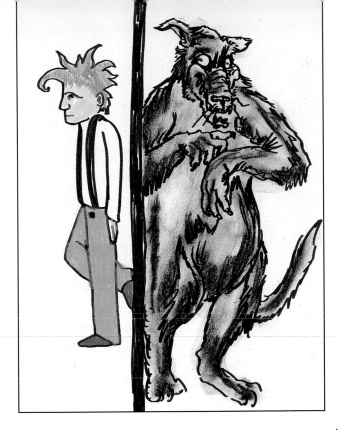

The most important thing to remember about depression and the beast is that . . . You and the beast are not the same, you are two separate beings. It's perfectly clear it's not your fault nor is it a character flaw.

You are you!
And the beast is depression.

The first question you ask is Why me? You may be feeling you did something wrong... Like you're being punished.

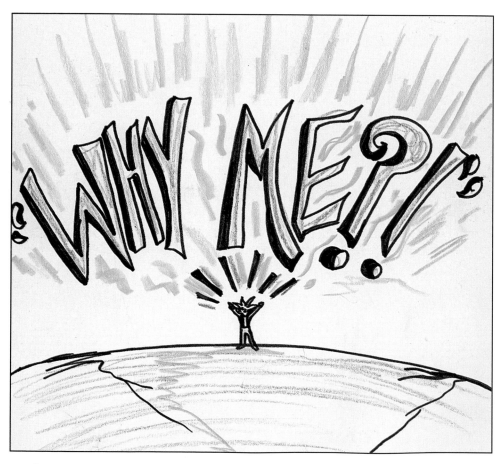

The reality is you didn't do anything wrong but it's tough to believe it.

I asked the question "Why me?" many times, but you have to realize it's not a punishment and you don't deserve it.

I t's an illness just like the flu and you don't have control over getting it. But society tends to look at mental illness differently from physical illness.

N O T E :

Depression is not a

weakness, it's an

illness that's curable.

The "beauty" of depression is there's so much more to gain than lose from the experience.

The feeling you'll get when you face and defeat the beast is worth the fight. When your battle is won you'll be able to face anything on the horizon.

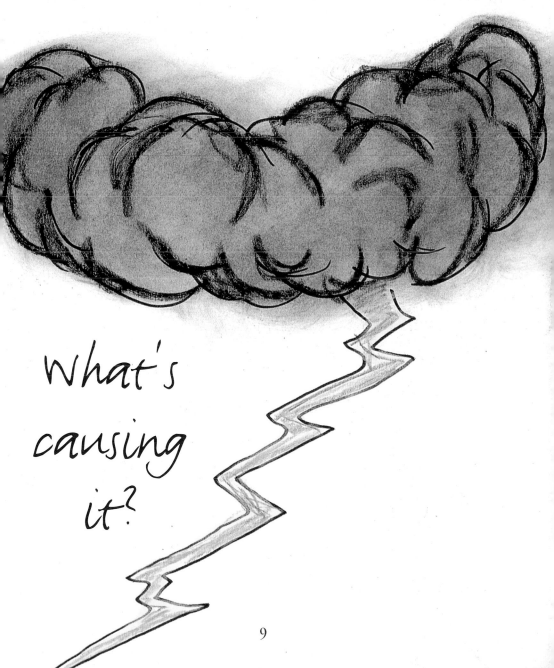

So, you're depressed? Why does it feel so out of control?

What's causing it?

9

When I first found out I was depressed, I kept wondering when did it start? Then it hit me, I had been depressed for about a year. The reason I didn't notice it before was because in the beginning the illness starts out small. I thought nothing about it, perhaps a bad day, and I accepted it because I thought it was part of my life. But it grew rapidly. The sadness became deep and went on unstoppable for weeks. It was growing inside of me and got big before I realized something was seriously wrong.

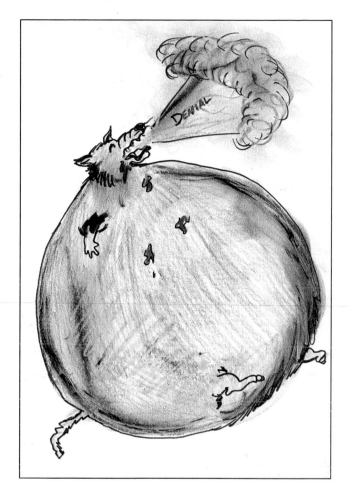

The beast had consumed me. I didn't want to admit it so I kept it inside and kept denying that something was wrong. It was as though I had invited him to an "all you can eat buffet."

soon he
grew...

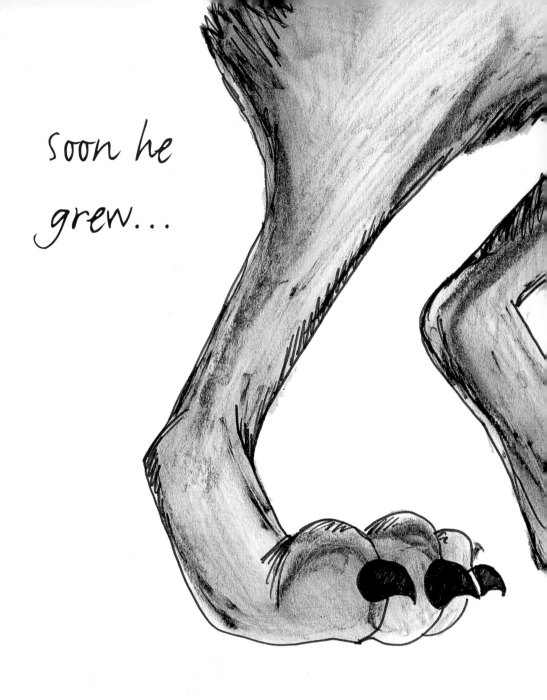

out of control...to a point
where I couldn't handle it.

The beast can't stand positive feelings that are really there, like understanding, love and trust, etc. He consumes them, leaving you with negative ones like paranoia, hopelessness and especially no trust.

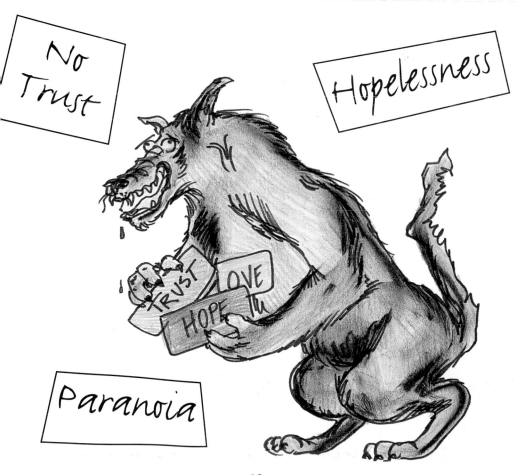

Trust is the beast's favorite meal,

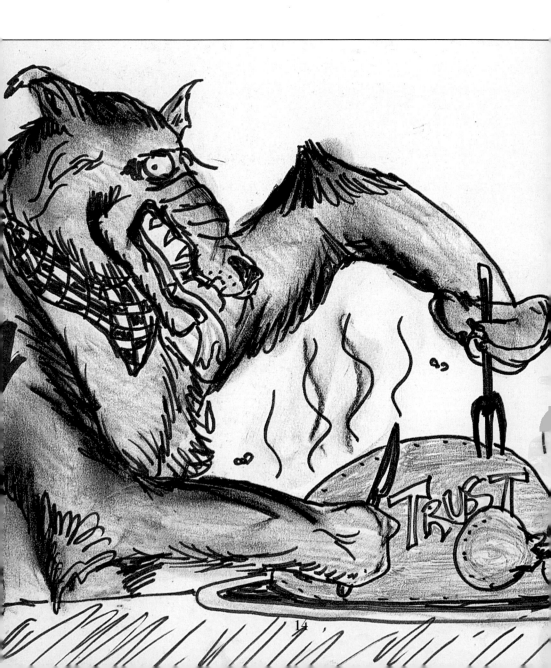

Trust is so important and it's terrible when you lose it. When I lost it I couldn't even trust my family, much less my friends. I always felt they thought I was a burden and that they were talking about me. Remember, that insecurity is part of the illness. Maybe a picture will explain.

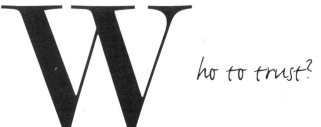

W ho to trust?

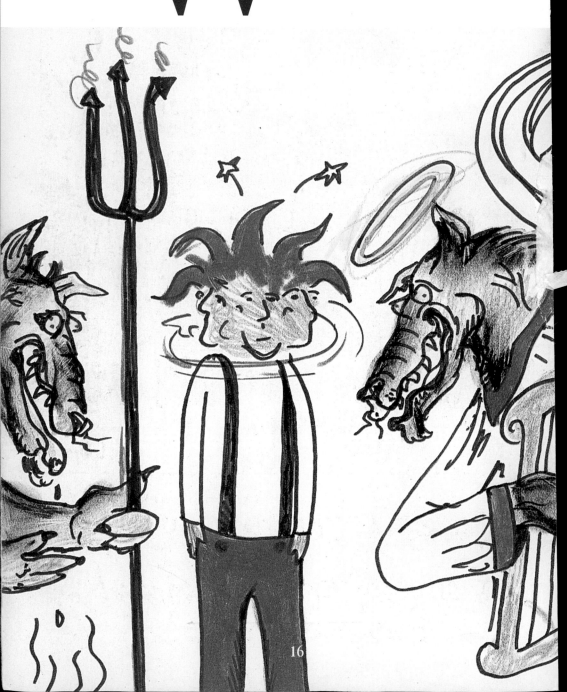

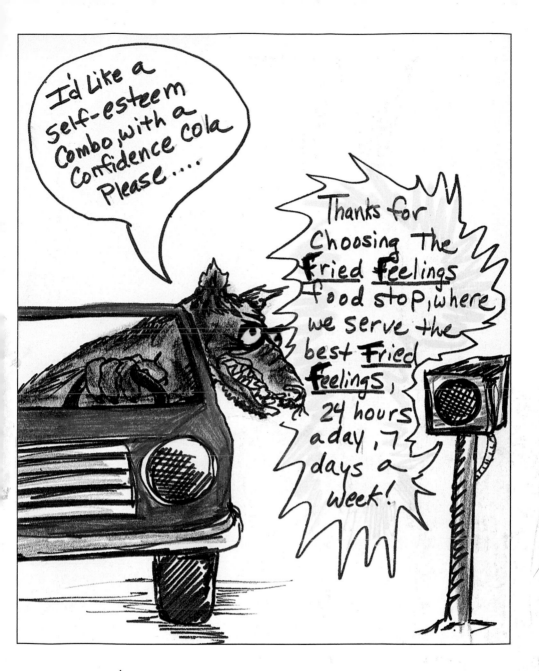

He begins feasting on your
self-esteem and Confidence...

Then happiness...

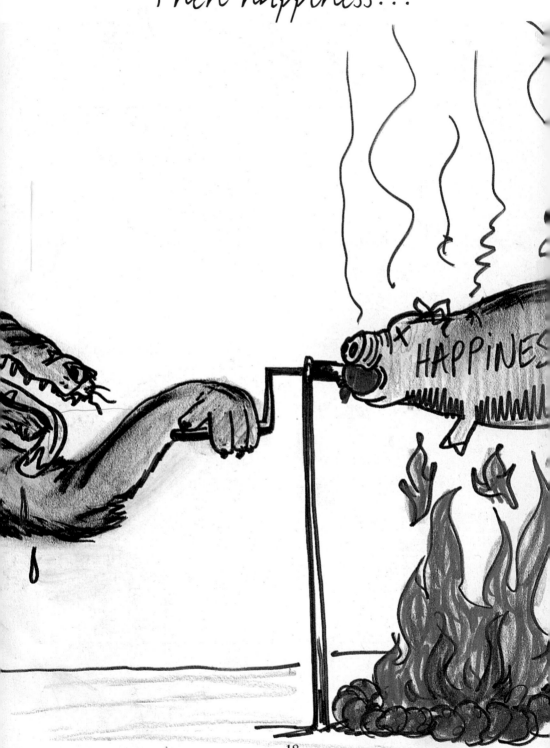

Next he feeds on your pride and dignity

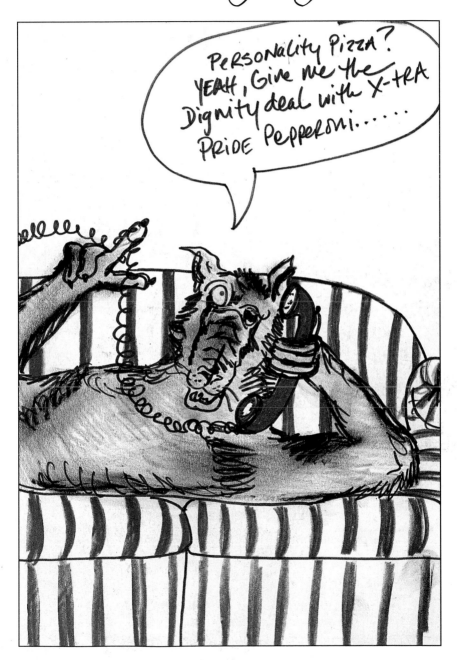

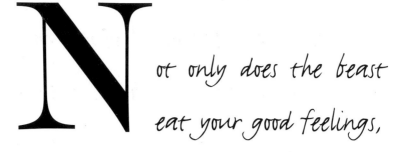

N ot only does the beast eat your good feelings,

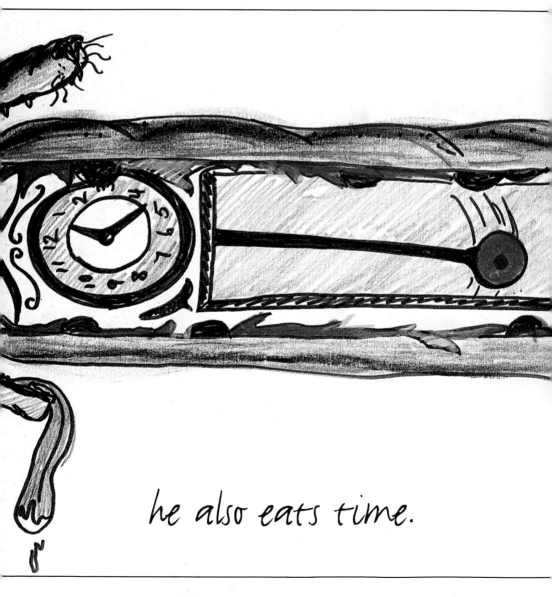

he also eats time.

There are other bad feelings that are running through your head and sometimes they're out of control. Feelings like anger... You might take it out on other people... When really you're angry at the beast.

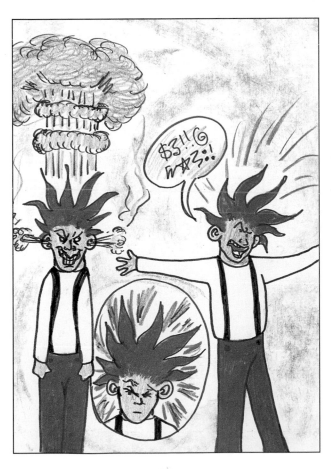

CHAPTER TWO

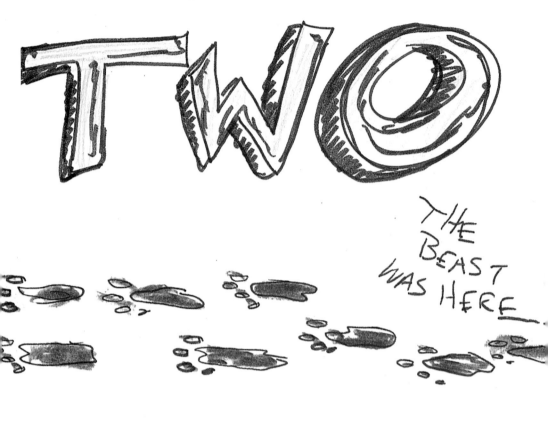

THE BEAST WAS HERE

SYMPTOMS OF THE BEAST

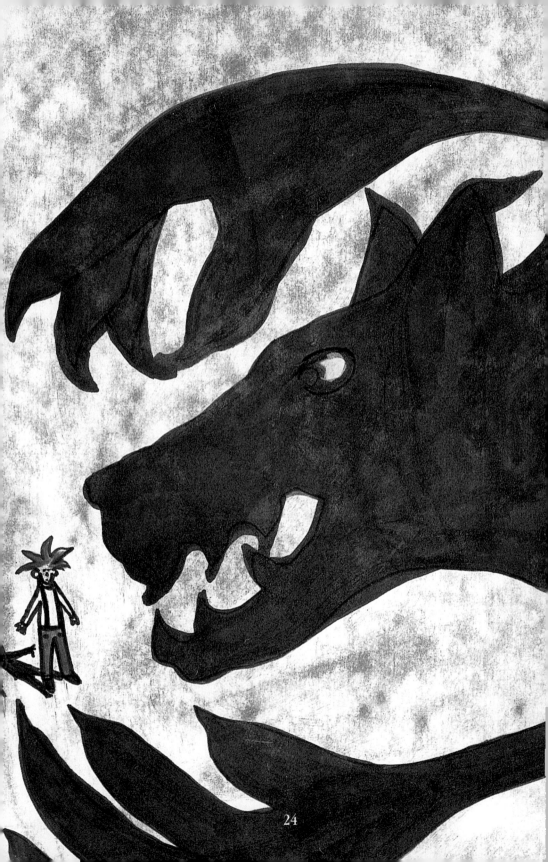

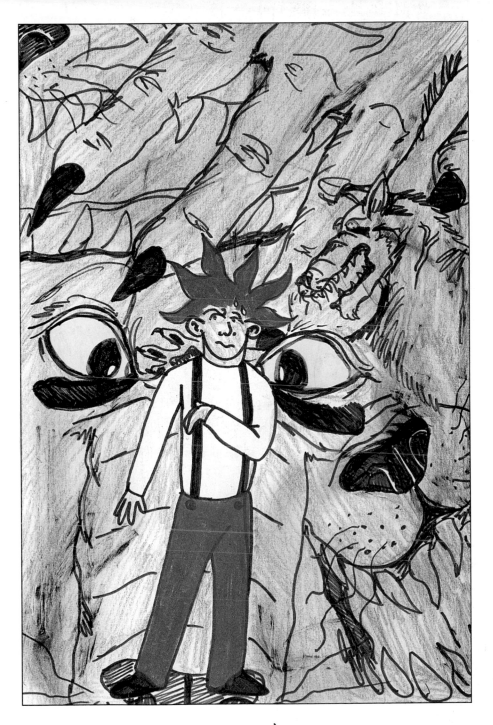

Paranoia.....

sadness...Loneliness...

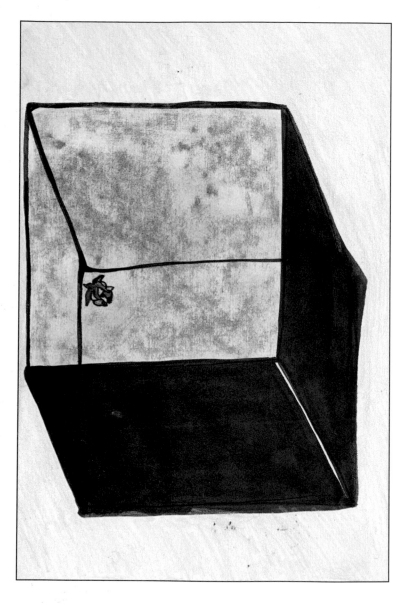

You might start to feel trapped.

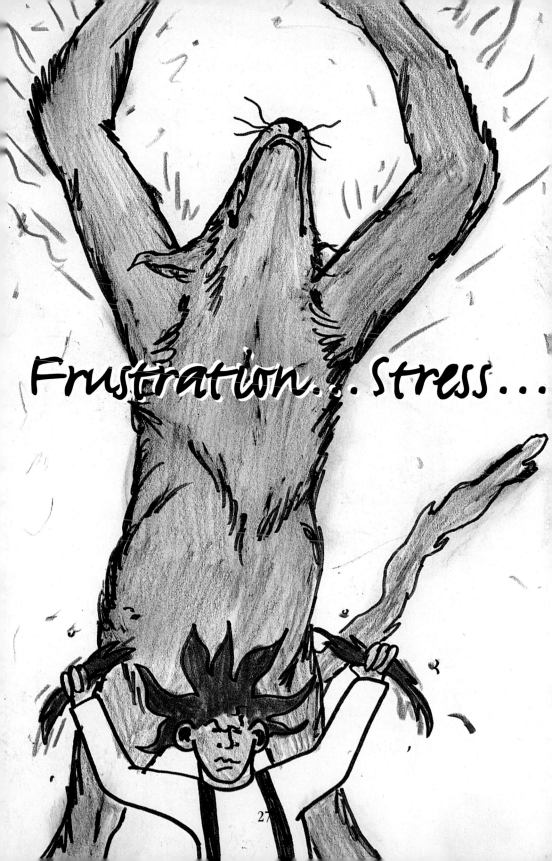

Frustration... Stress...

Sometimes you can't see the real you.

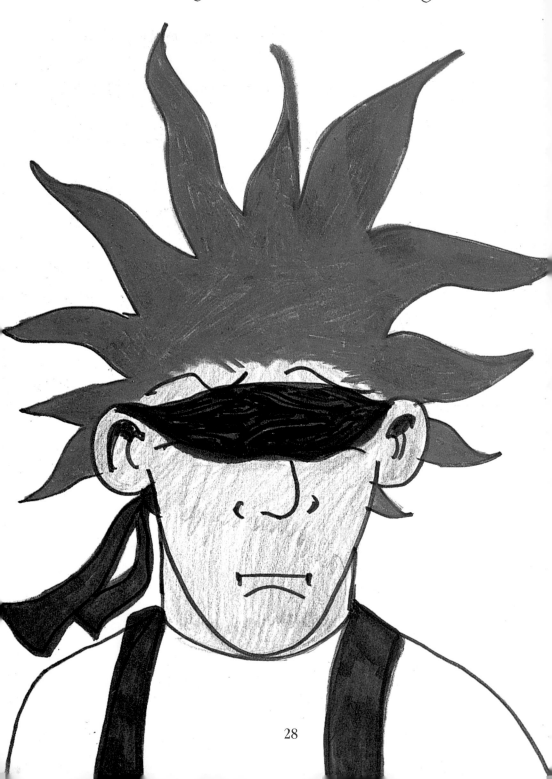

28

Inside, you could have everything that it takes to make yourself really happy, but the beast has taken **everything** from you, leaving you totally depressed.

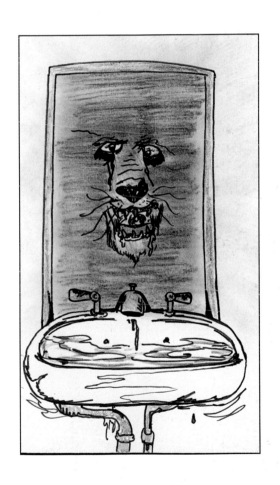

All **you** can see is ...him.

T

he beast blinds you from many things like...

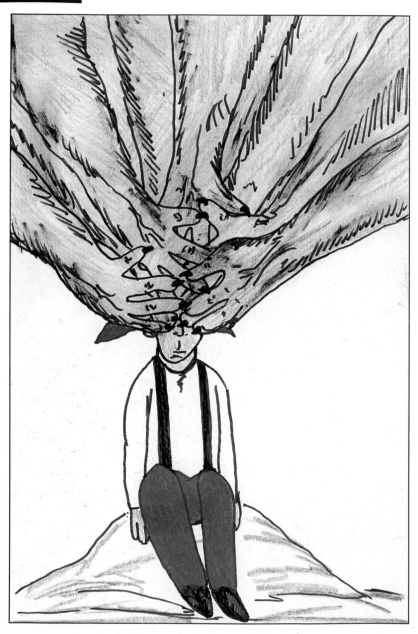

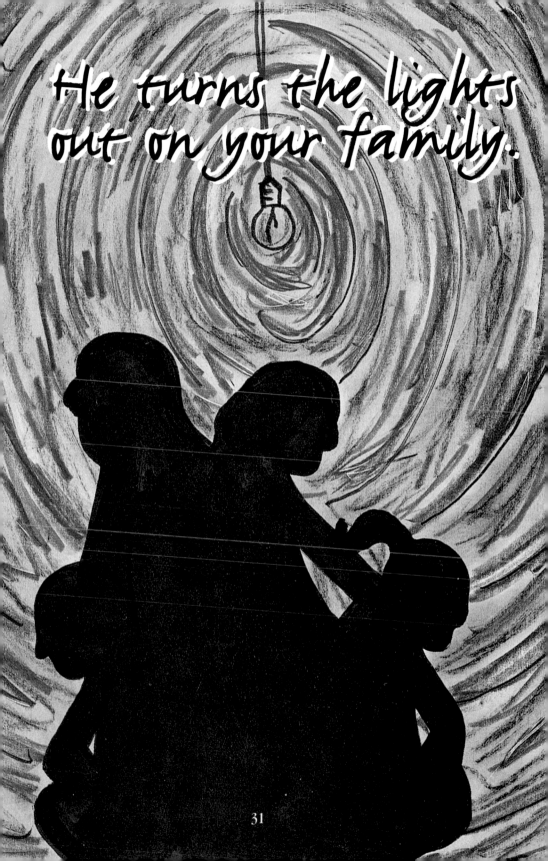

He turns the lights out on your family.

31

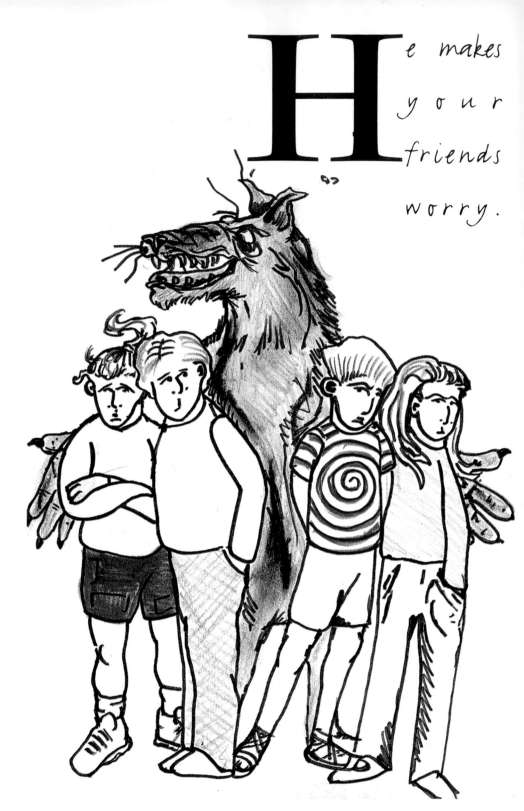

H e makes your friends worry.

Family and friends are very important, but sometimes they don't understand because they may also be confused and scared.

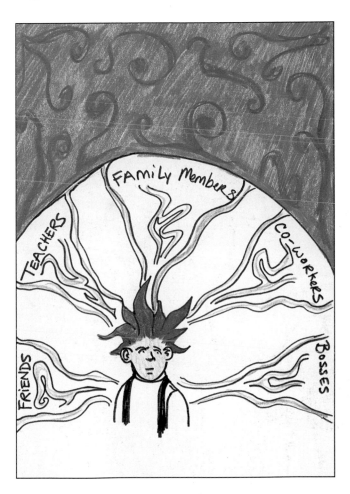

When you're depressed it confuses everyone around you.

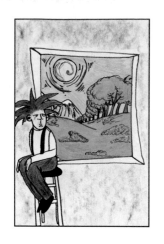

Sometimes depression can affect you physically, like me. I had all the symptoms, such as...

Always feeling tired and weak. You don't have any drive or ambition, nothing matters, no matter how important it is.

Some days you don't even want to leave your room.

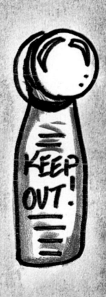

Your eating habits might change as well. I lost a lot of weight and it felt terrible! You might find yourself eating too much or not wanting to eat at all. I experienced many other symptoms, too. Such as...

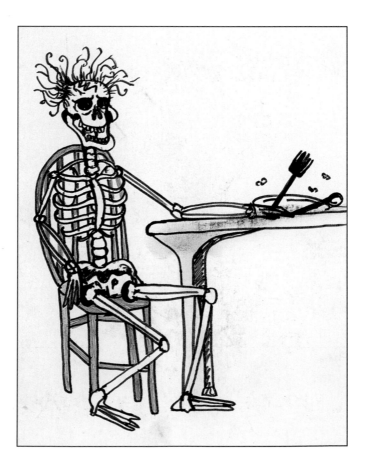

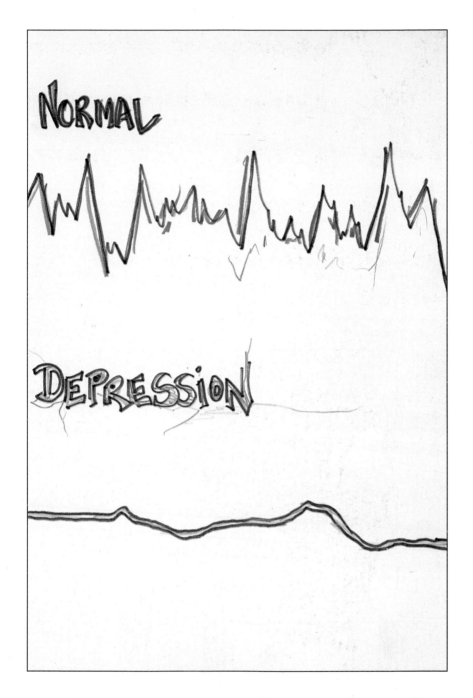

slurred or slow speech

Blurred 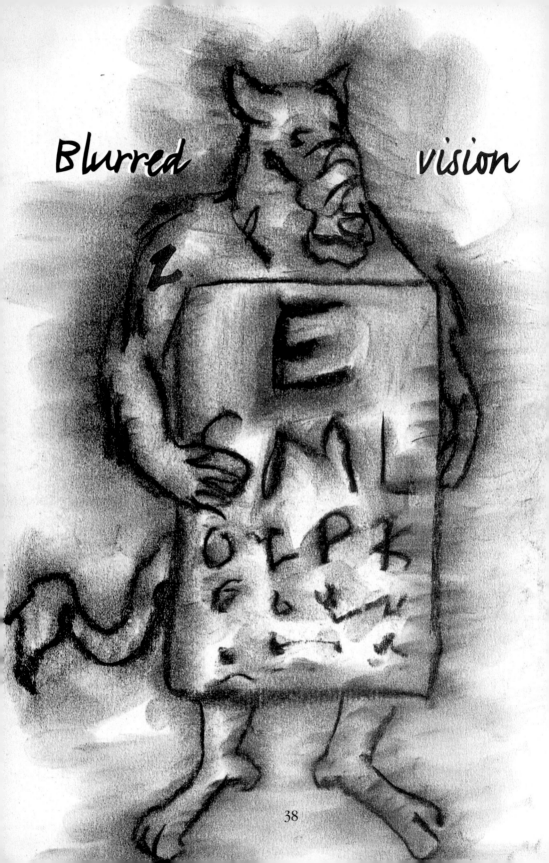 vision

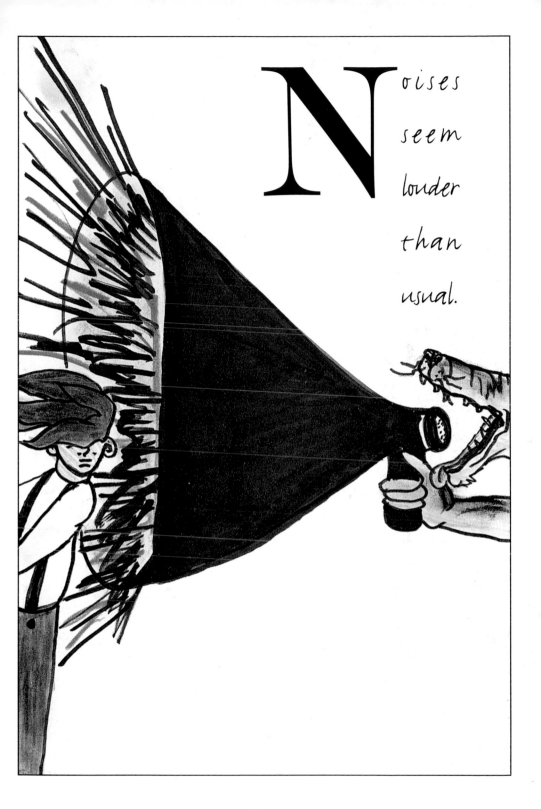

N oises seem louder than usual.

Headaches

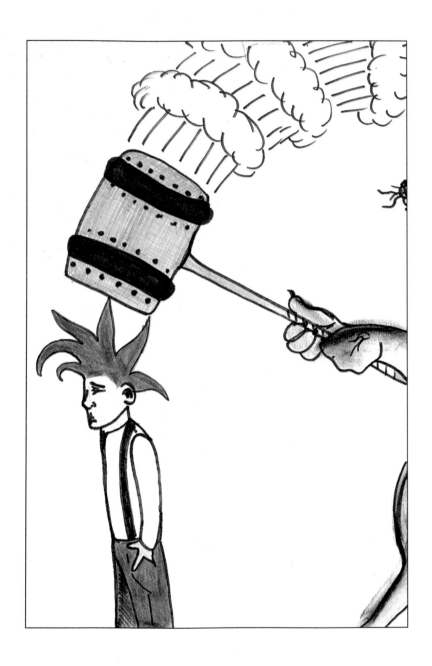

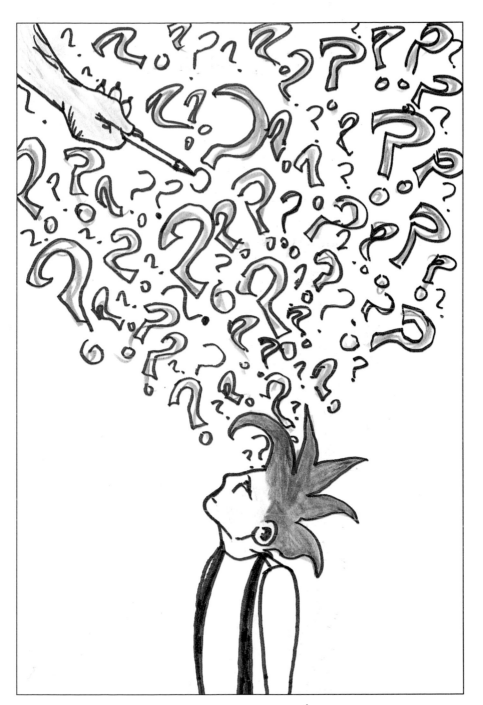

Memory loss

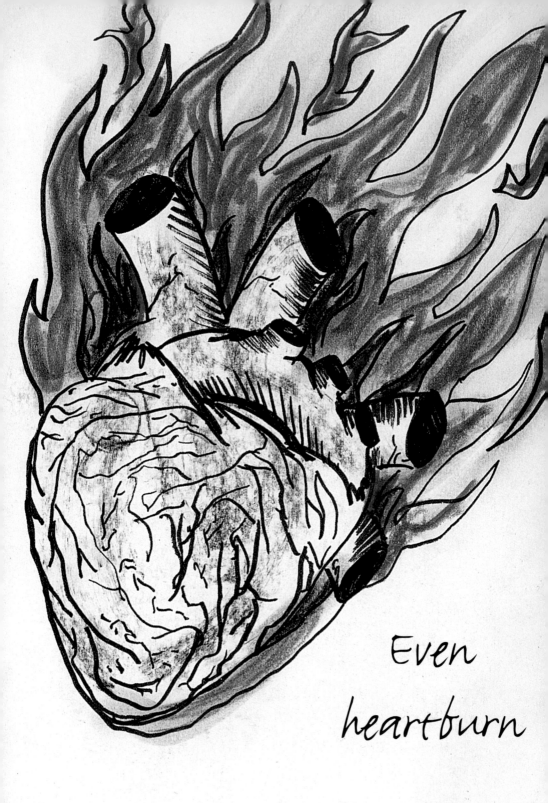

Even

heartburn

42

The beast sometimes makes it impossible to fall asleep.

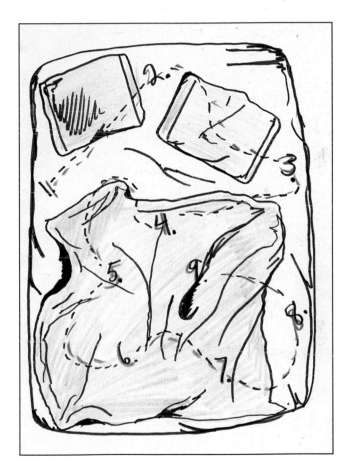

When you finally do fall asleep you have won the battle but the war may have just begun.

The war comes in the form of nightmares

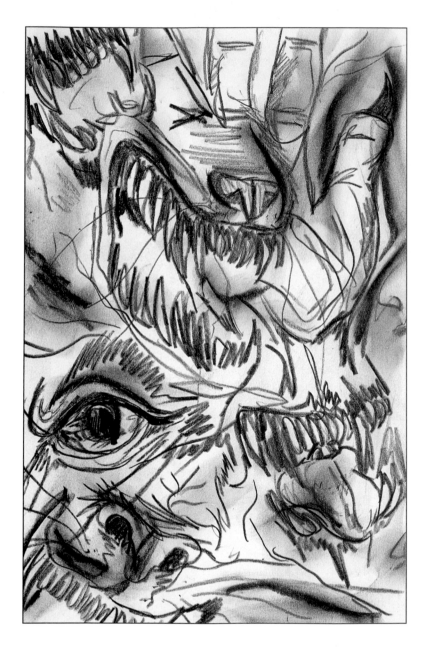

one right after another. . . . Night after night.

M
any times people lose hope.

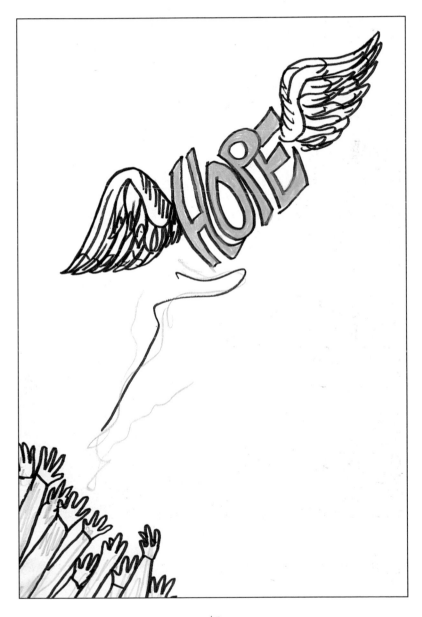

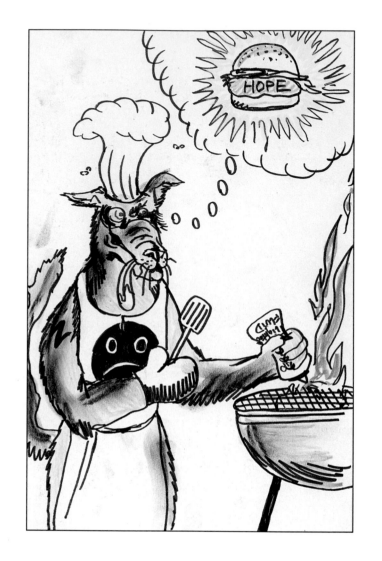

With hope all things are possible. Without hope the beast easily wins. That's why barbecuing Hope burgers is his specialty.

CHAPTER

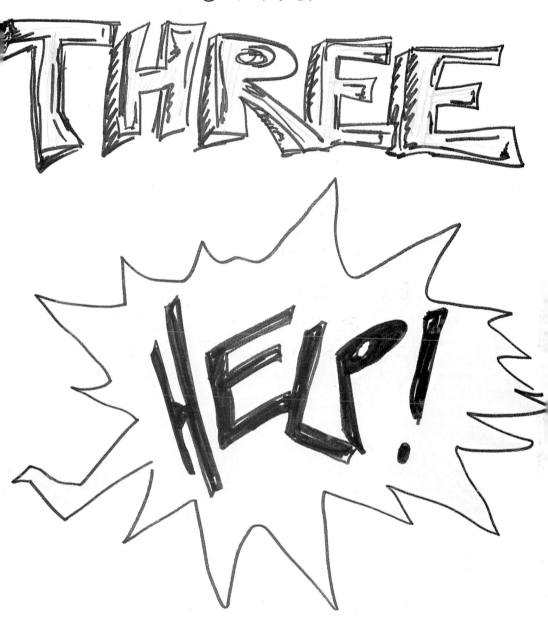

THREE

HELP!

ASK FOR HELP

Rather than ask for help, a lot of times kids try to help themselves.

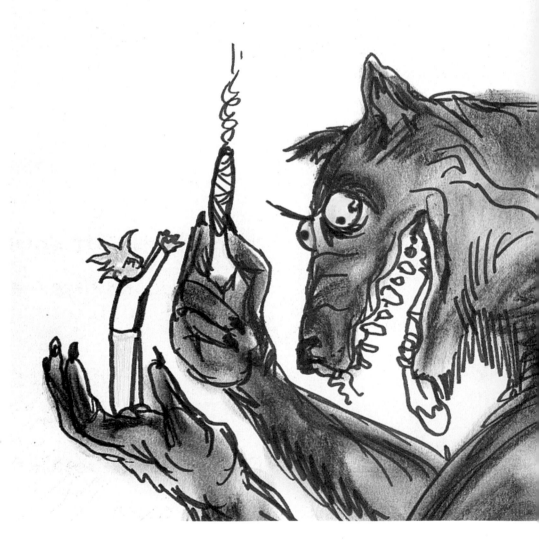

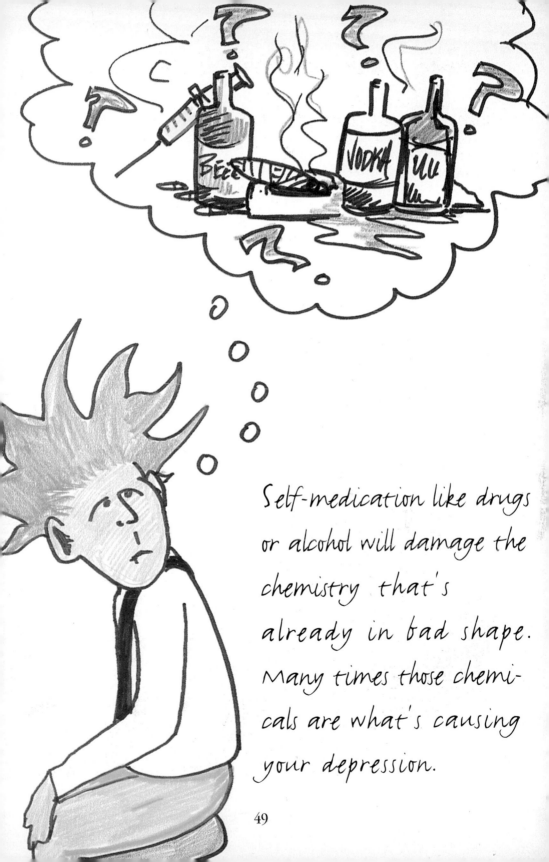

Self-medication like drugs or alcohol will damage the chemistry that's already in bad shape. Many times those chemicals are what's causing your depression.

49

The worst thing you could ever do is think that suicide is the ultimate self-help.

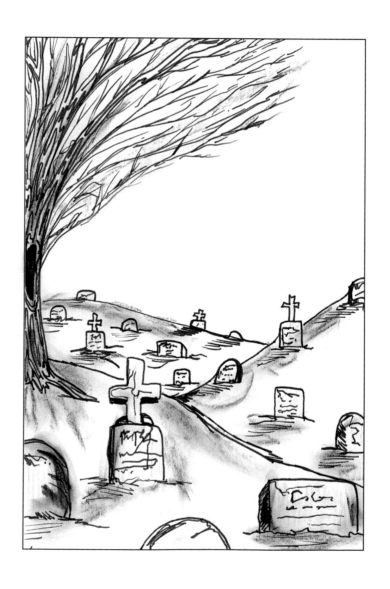

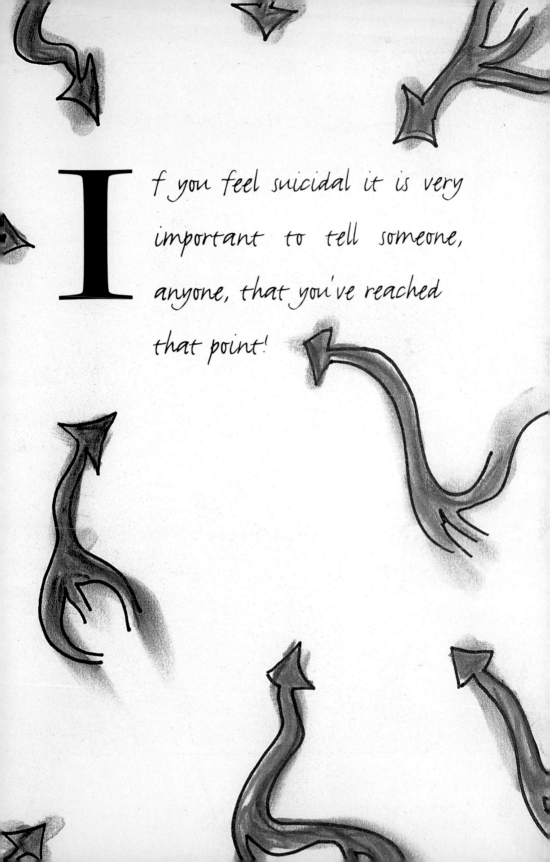

If you feel suicidal it is very important to tell someone, anyone, that you've reached that point!

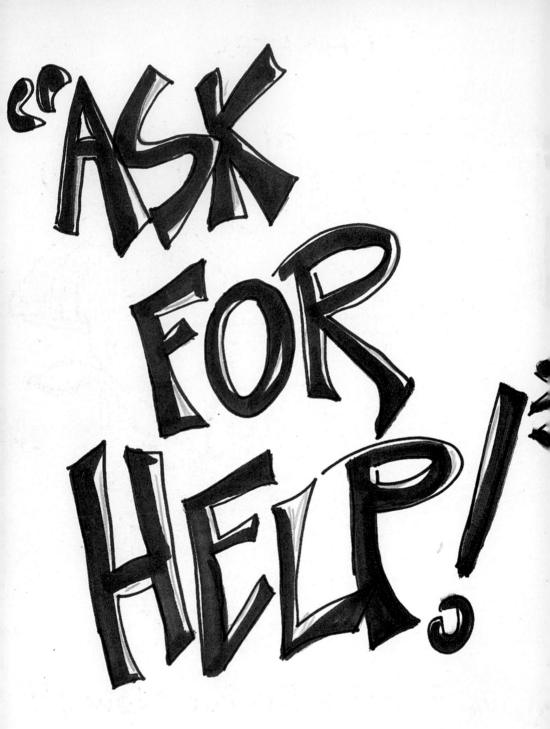

"ASK FOR HELP!

(Helplines are included on page 101)

CHAPTER

FOUR

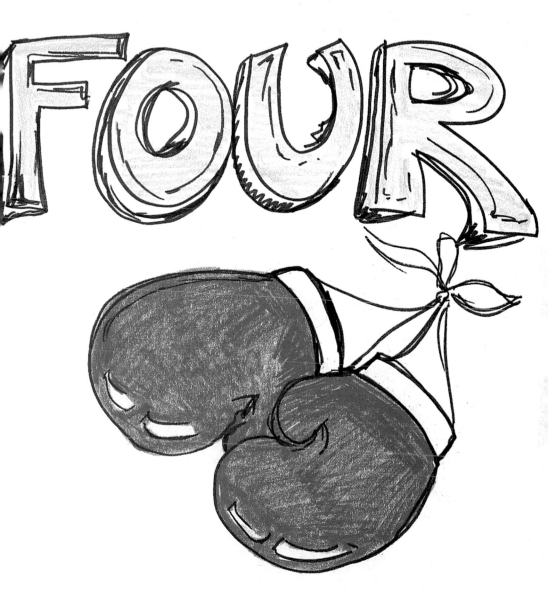

YOUR BATTLE BEGINS NOW !!!

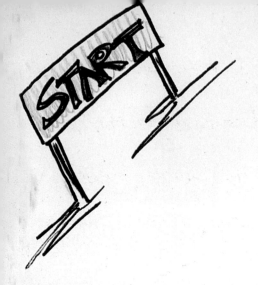

As soon as you start to get help the struggle with your beast will begin. Be ready to fight hard because you are the only one who can shrink him. Here are some ways that will help you out.

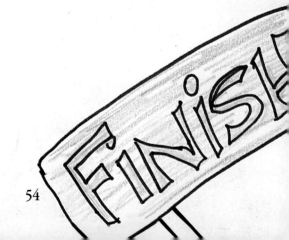

Your battle will be extremely scary, but you'll find courage you thought you never had once you've made the commitment to fight.

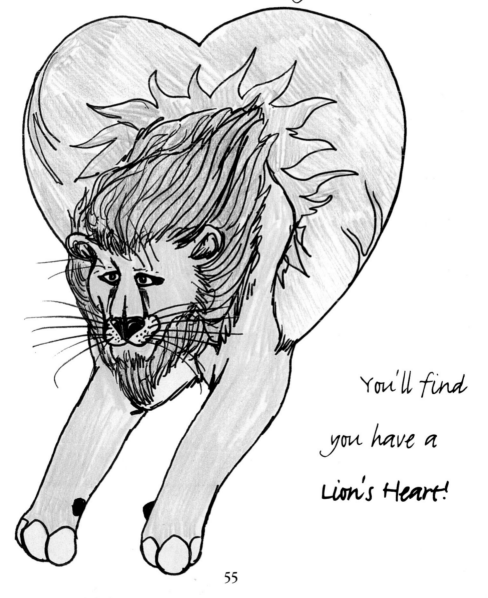

You'll find you have a **Lion's Heart!**

The first thing to do is talk to someone like a friend, a counselor, family member or clergy. A counselor is probably your best bet. If you're young like me it's good to talk to your mom and dad. If they're not available, talk to a close adult friend who cares about you.

Counseling is a great start but the beast hates it because he knows it will help you. So he plugs his ears. You may need more help, like medicine.

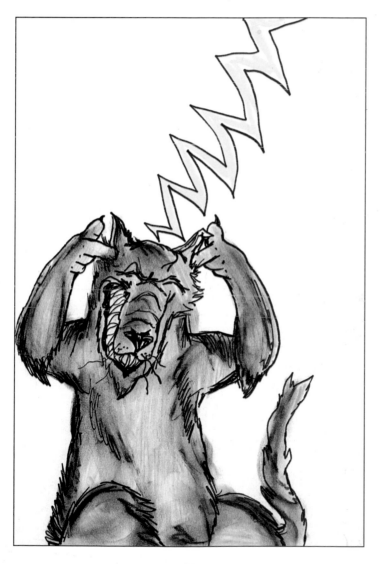

57

Medicine can help get your body chemistry back on track, but he will do everything he can to flush your medicine down the toilet.

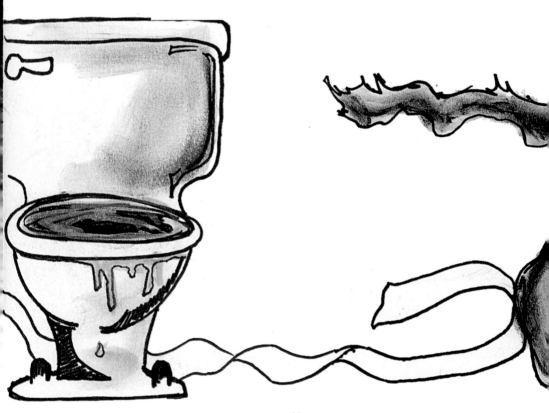

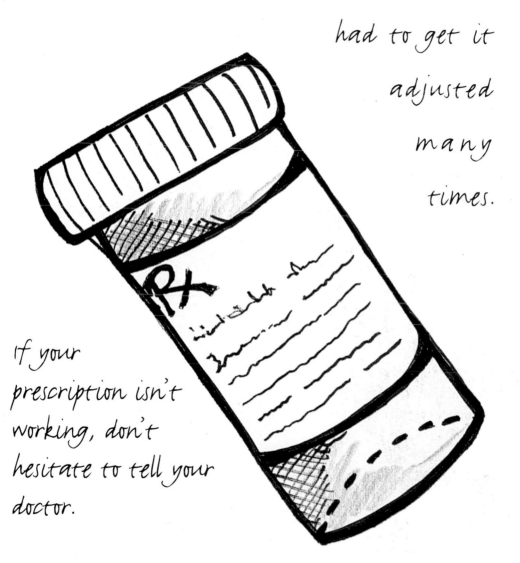

Sometimes when you take medicine to balance out the chemicals in your brain, it might not work. So it might have to be changed. With me, I had to get it adjusted many times.

If your prescription isn't working, don't hesitate to tell your doctor.

S

ee, medicine is like poison to the beast. When he's hungry he'll go for a slab of feelings.

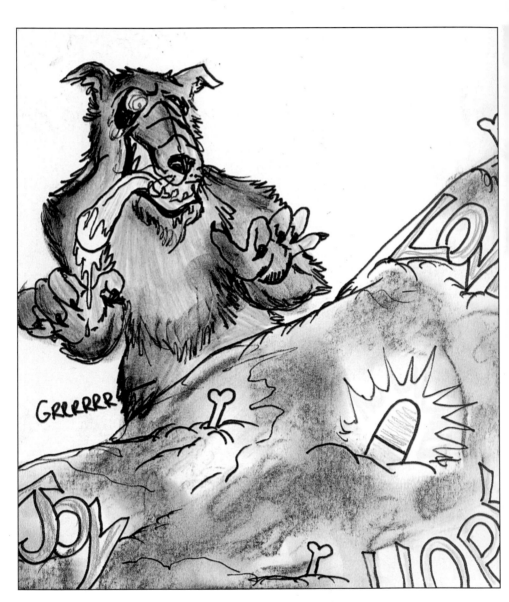

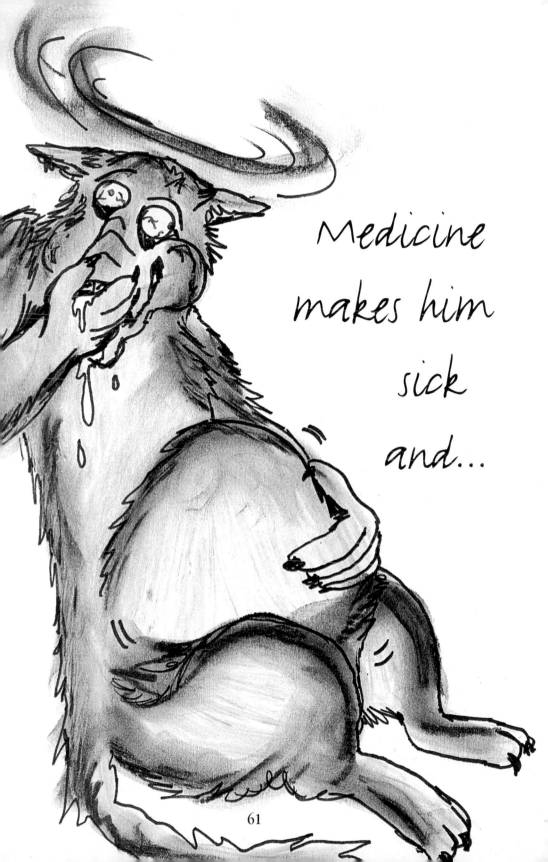

Medicine

makes him

sick

and...

61

Mad

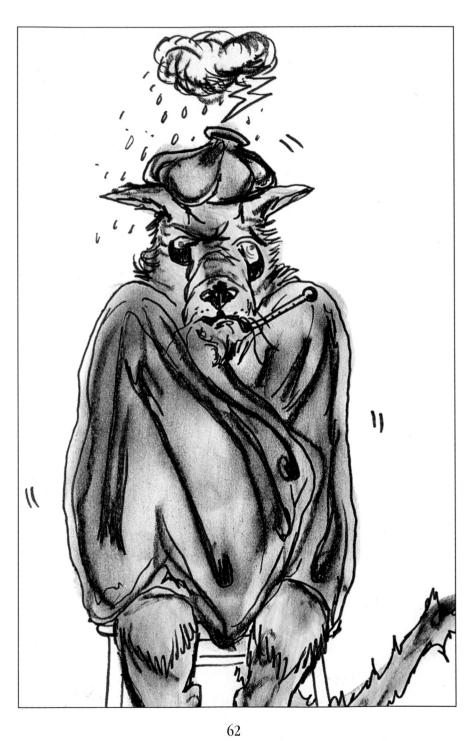

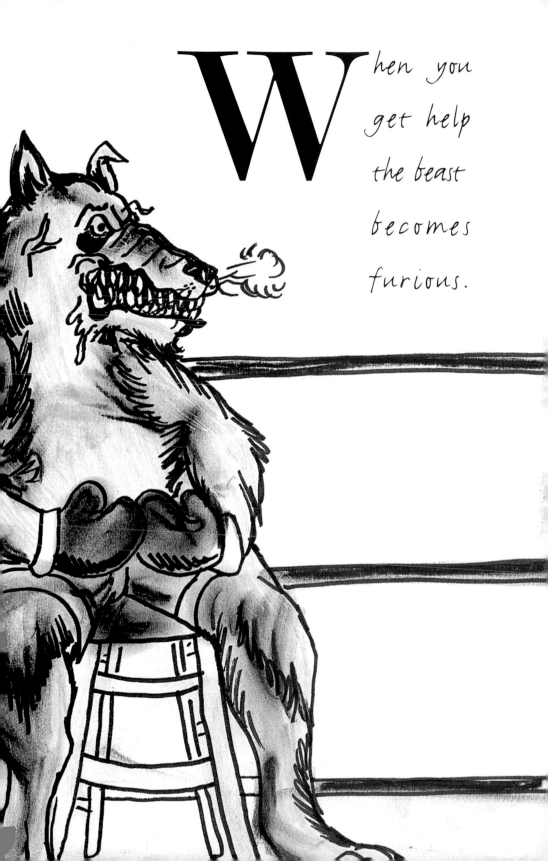

When you get help the beast becomes furious.

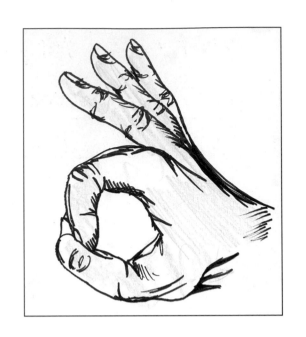

He fights hard, sometimes too hard. sometimes you might need a little more to shrink him down to size. It may take a higher dosage of medicine. If your beast is still unstoppable, you might need to go to the hospital for a little while. That's ok, just keep thinking about what will help you and what will shrink your beast.

A lot of times I felt discouraged when my medicine had to be changed so much. You will have times when you fall down on your climb to mental wellness. Don't worry. It doesn't mean you're going to be so bad off again. Be prepared. Do things you like ... things that make you happy; that give you an extra burst of courage or that fill those empty spaces in you. Things like...

65

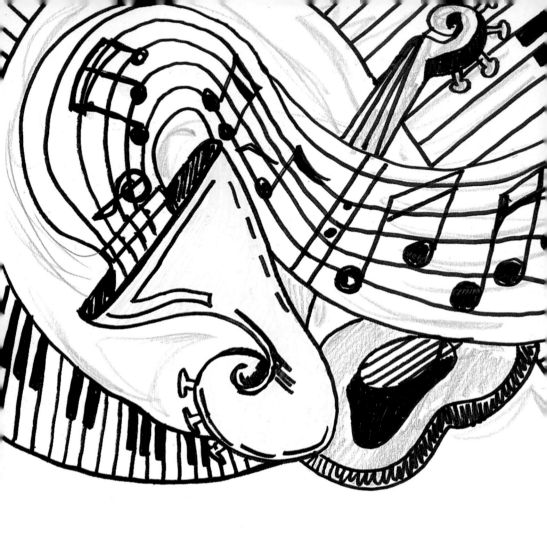

Music played a key role in my recovery. Listen to whatever music helps **you** the most.

Watching a good TV show usually helps, too. It was always calming for me to go to a movie because it is quiet and peaceful.

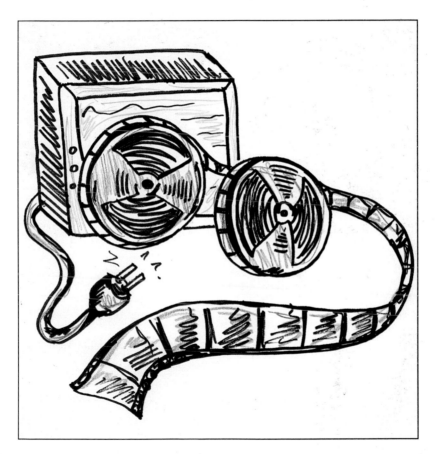

You can escape and get your mind off of your problems for a while.

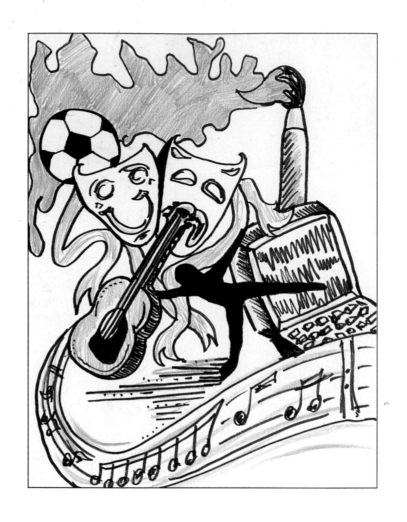

One thing that helps is to find a hobby, something that you're good at and love doing. A hobby can help pull you through. For me it was art. As a matter of fact writing this book helped me get through my battle.

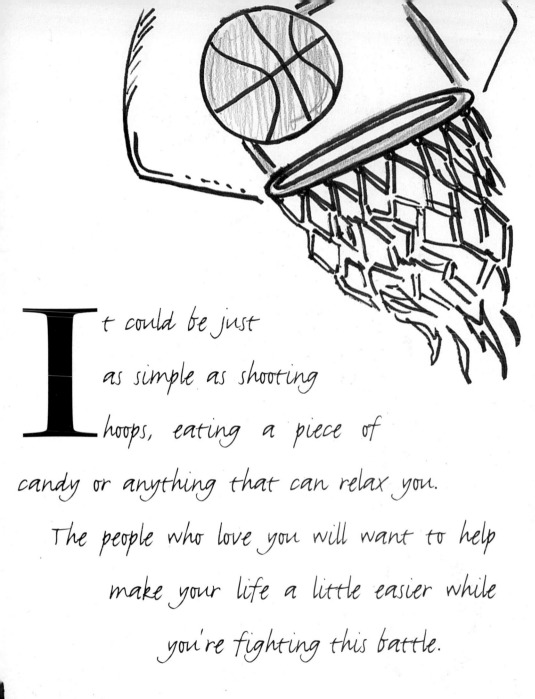

I t could be just
as simple as shooting
hoops, eating a piece of
candy or anything that can relax you.
   The people who love you will want to help
      make your life a little easier while
         you're fighting this battle.

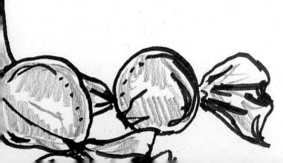

I

t could be going to
the zoo, or being out
in nature.

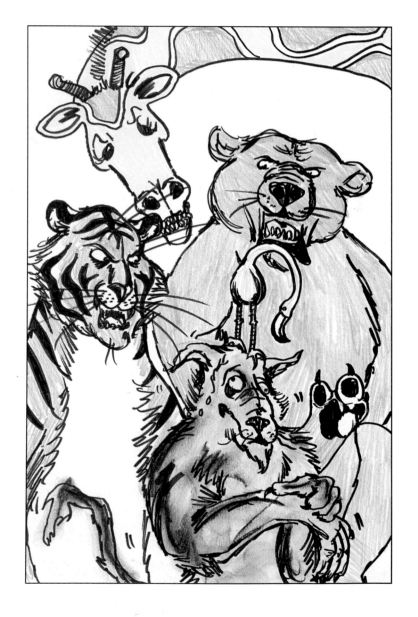

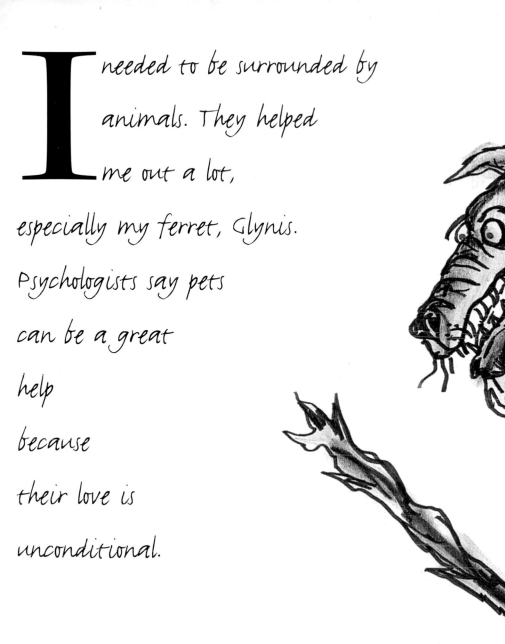

I needed to be surrounded by animals. They helped me out a lot, especially my ferret, Glynis. Psychologists say pets can be a great help because their love is unconditional.

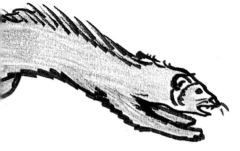

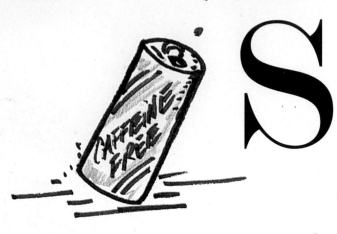

Some ways that you can help yourself physically are...

Less sugar intake. That was tough because I love sugar. It's also good to get some vitamins, especially if you have problems with eating. Check your local health food stores.

Eat foods with high protein, like beans! Ahhhhh! They doooo taste good in a bean burrito at Taco Bell.

Exercise. Yes, it's hard. So start out slow then gradually build up.

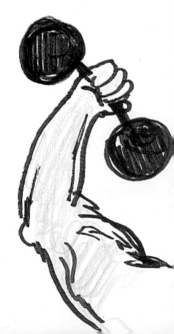

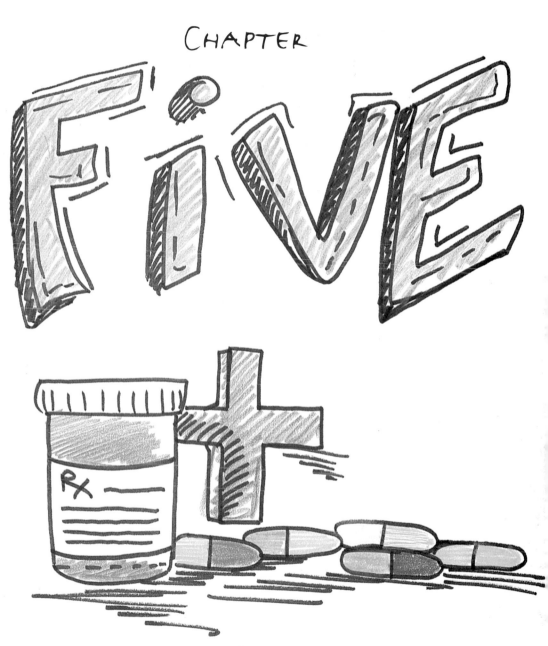

CHAPTER

FiVE

THERAPY, HOSPITALIZATION
AND HEALING

If you have to go to the hospital it will be scary at first, especially if you don't know what's going to happen. I'll tell you what happened to me. It may vary in some ways from hospital to hospital.

The reason that I needed to check into the hospital was that I got to a point when I couldn't trust myself. I didn't know if I wanted to live or die. I went to the hospital to talk about my problems and to find the right medicine to help me. But most importantly to keep me safe.

When I arrived at the hospital it was really hard to be left there. But before my mom left, we worked out a plan for phone calls. The hospital had to approve it to make sure the people I talked to were a good influence.

I was allowed two calls in the morning and two at night. I found a lot of inner courage experiencing this. My mom brought me some things from home, like my pillow and my favorite stuffed animal. The hospital staff checked everything for items which I could use to hurt myself. I got a routine check-up by the doctor who took my weight, blood pressure and all the basics.

The first night I was in there was hard. The room didn't have anything in it except a bathroom, bed and some drawers. The next morning I had to get up bright and early. The food wasn't all that hot. The staff went over the daily schedule. Then came the hard part. A total physical. That day was probably the hardest day of all because I thought I had taken every test in the book. In the hospital I received information on the various levels of progression through their program. The more my condition improved, the more freedom I received.

Here are the levels:

1) Suicide and escape precautions	3) Level Three - more privileges
2) Level two - still pretty strict	4) Level four - freedom

When you get on level four you're almost ready to go home. At first my family could only visit me for a couple of hours during the week and on weekends. The more the staff got to know me, the more I considered them as friends, rather than superiors. I had a roommate that had already been through the system so that helped.

W hen I was released from the hospital I became discouraged very easily because I felt vulnerable. I felt a lot of pressure to be the enthusiastic person I once was...the actor, the athlete.

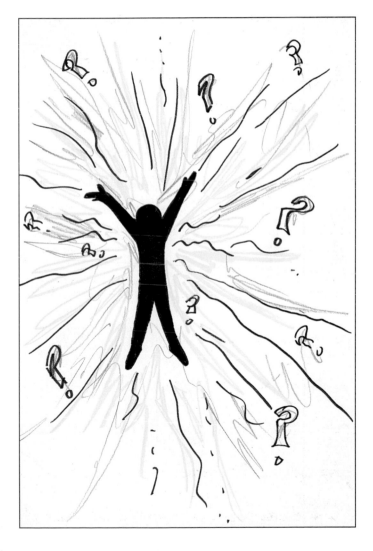

I had to keep on going to counseling and it's hard spilling your guts to doctor after doctor, but you've got to stick with it because medicine alone won't cure you.

You have to be

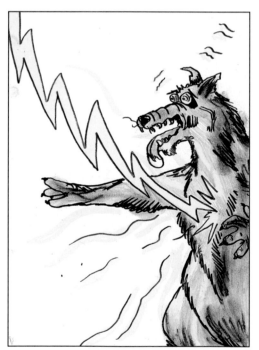

BIG and BRAVE!

The counseling will help shrink your beast.

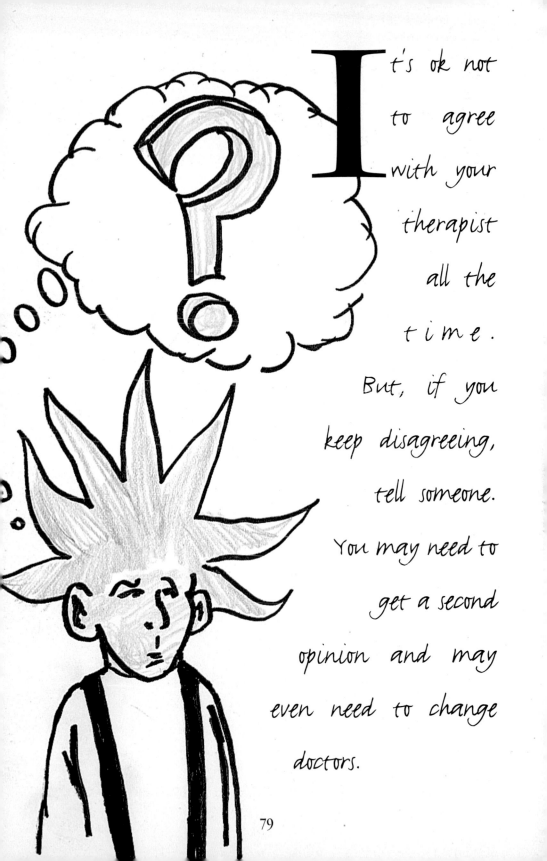

It's ok not to agree with your therapist all the time. But, if you keep disagreeing, tell someone. You may need to get a second opinion and may even need to change doctors.

We started to see a pattern within my depressive behavior. PMS symptoms and depression symptoms are almost identical. My hormone levels seemed to be making my depression twice as bad, once a month. That's the last thing you need to deal with! Talk to your therapist or psychiatrist about seeing a gynecologist. I know it's another doctor to see, but it might really help. It helped me to start taking hormone pills. They didn't interfere with my antidepressants.

CHAPTER Six

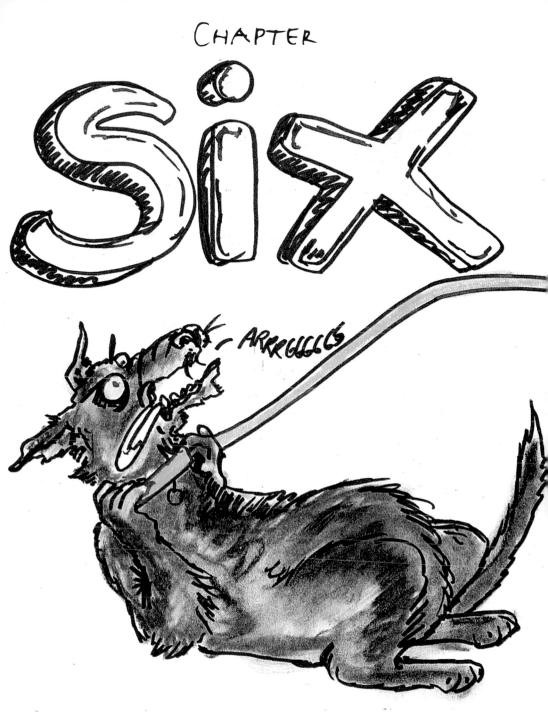

THE BEAST IS LEASHED

If you work hard enough, go to counseling, take your medicine and do the things that make you happy . . .

Then, you've got him on the run!

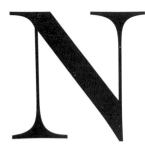 ext, you'll be able to put him on a leash.

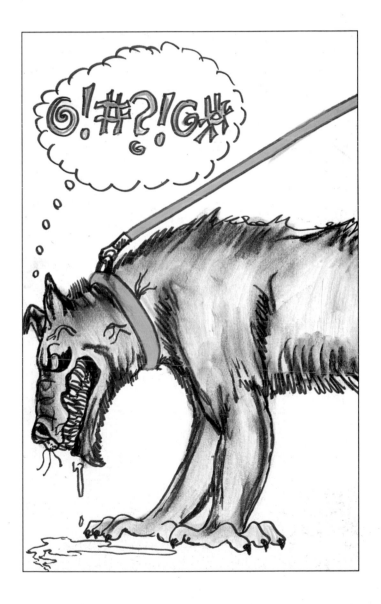

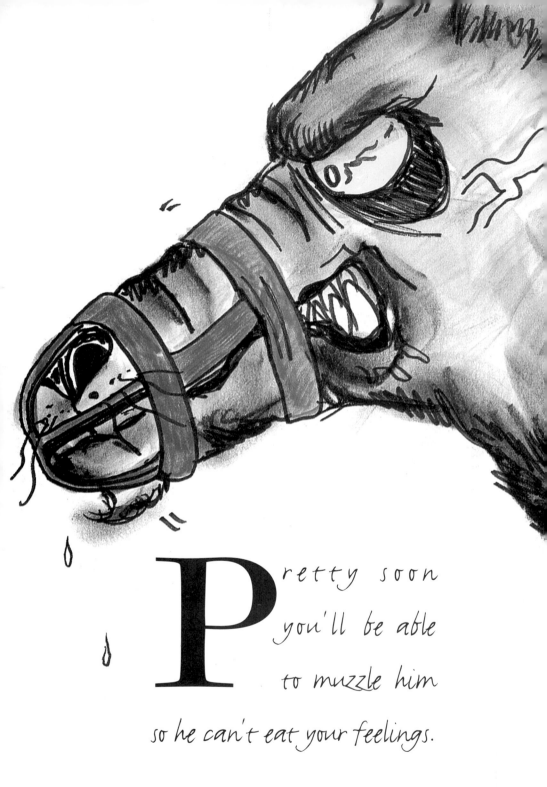

Pretty soon you'll be able to muzzle him so he can't eat your feelings.

Hey, how about a new look?

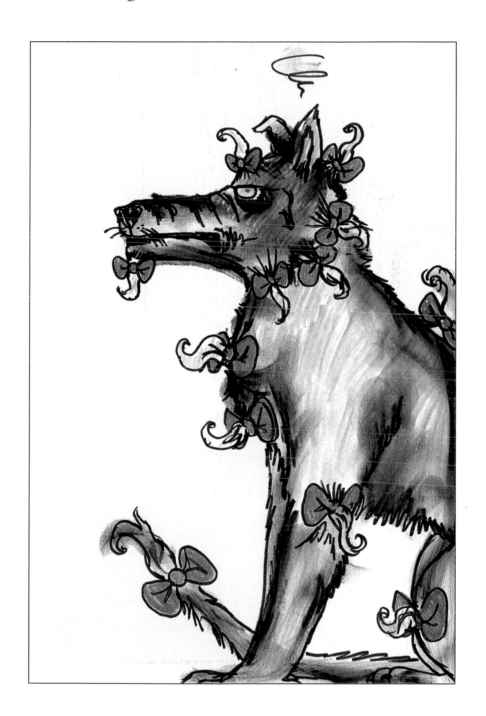

The more you keep fighting, the more you'll notice the beast starting to shrink! He doesn't like that very much. Too bad!

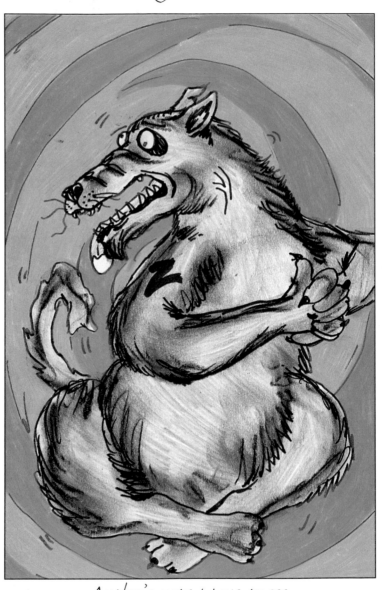

Author's note | Love to see the beast shrink, this can be so satisfying!

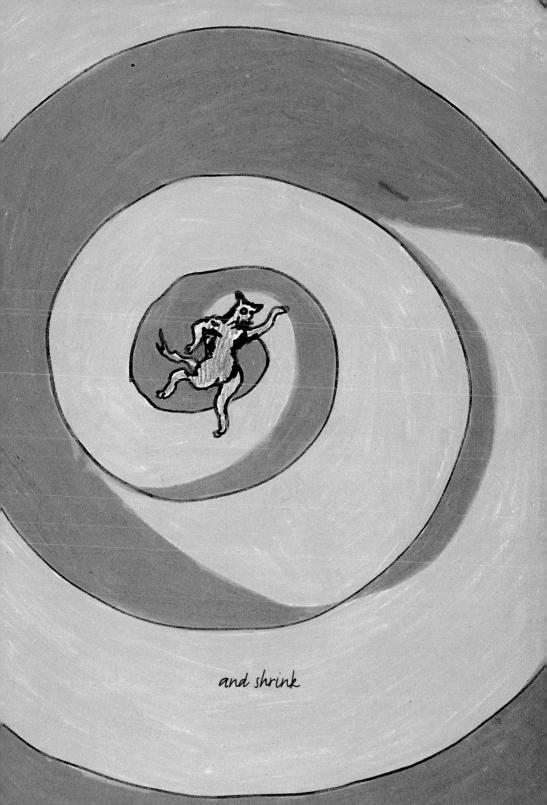

and shrink

87

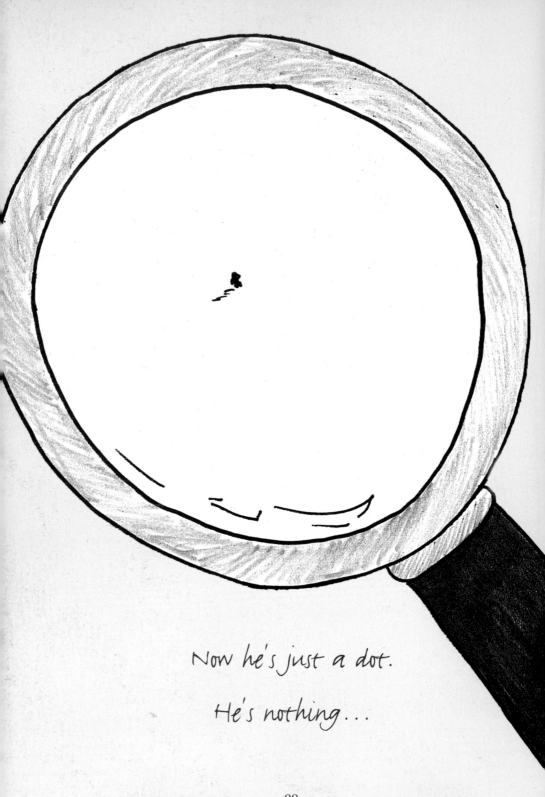

Now he's just a dot.

He's nothing...

As you begin to heal it's like going up a steep hill with some ups and downs.

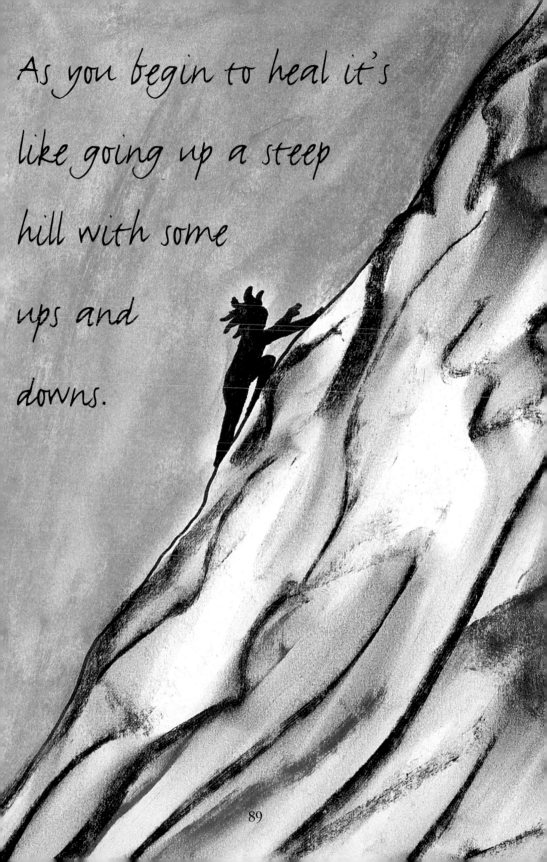

Sometimes you might have the feeling of being afraid to get better because it seems like when you get better there's too much to face or you won't get enough attention when you really need it.

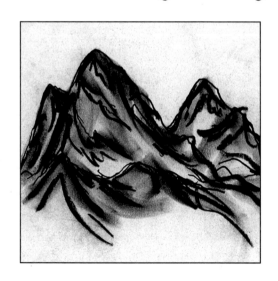

Don't worry. When you're better you will be so strong that you can face things that seem big and they'll be nothing. And the people that love you will always be there for you.

On your climb remember to take it slow, don't rush it. Stop and smell the roses and pet the mountain goat.

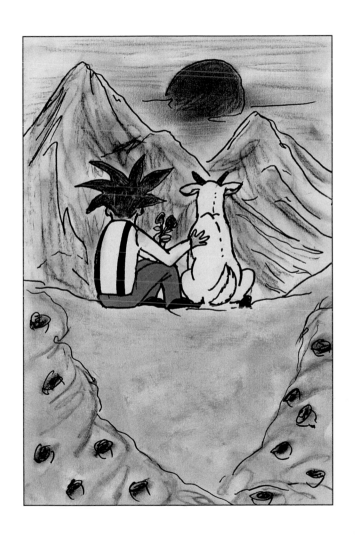

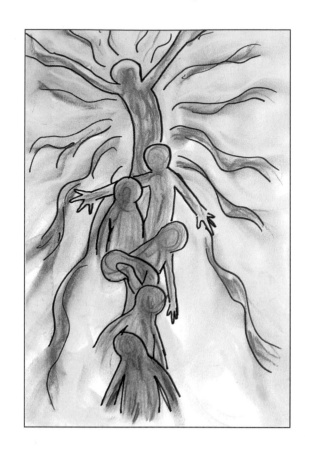

Y ou have gained your life back! For some strange but unbelievable reason a cat's fur feels softer, clouds make pictures like ferrets and every person, idea or thought makes your heart glow. You see things you've never noticed before...and it feels good!

The Road Map To Victory

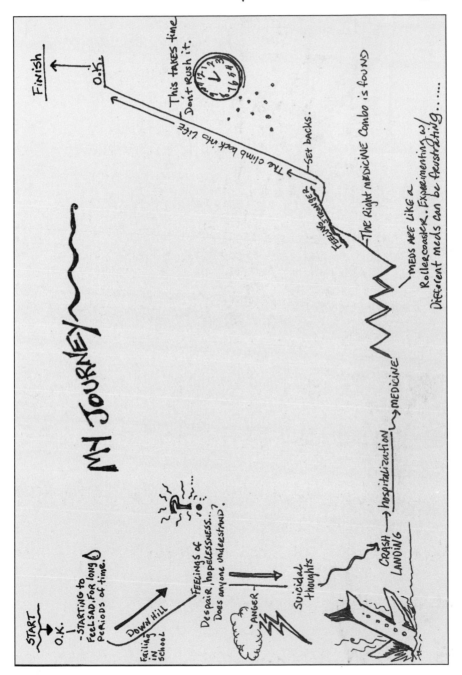

Now when you or someone you care about needs help you'll know what to do and say. You won't be afraid. You'll be full of courage, ready to challenge the beast...and win. I did and so can you.

Love,

Cait

Cait Irwin

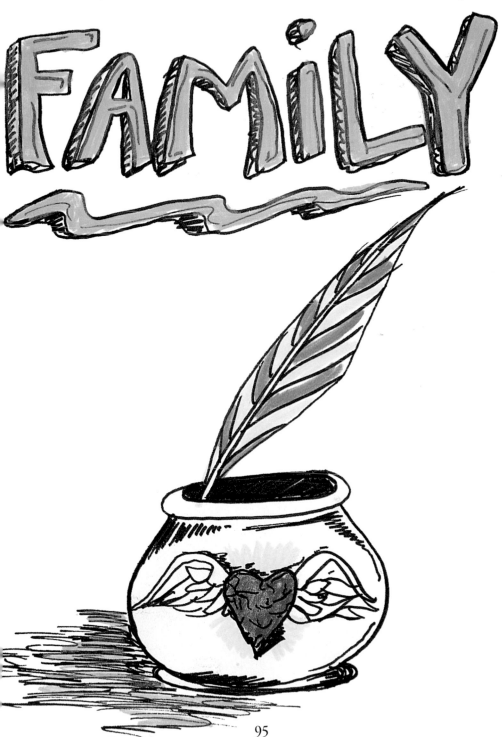

LETTERS FROM THE Family

A Letter from Cait's Mom

Dear Reader,

This could never happen to us . . . but it did. As close as we have always been, I was shocked to learn that Cait had put an artist's knife to her wrist the night before our first psychiatric appointment. If you, yourself, or someone you know is in the position of being the person to help a loved one suffering from depression, gather your courage and energy and begin to "challenge the beast."

You don't have to be an expert in psychology to begin to shrink the beast. You already have it in you, right now, to meet the challenge. To help someone who's depressed, here are some things I learned from the experience:

- Begin by recognizing that there is a problem. Take the initiative and follow Cait's advice in the book.
- Whatever you are now, start thinking of yourself as an *observer* so you can be a good *reporter* to the doctor, counselor, or teacher about what's happening. Keep a journal.

Be a positive *communicator* and *listener*. Make it clear you are committed to helping them to wellness. (Cait always asked me, "Are you going to give up on me?" I always answered, "Never.")

Be prepared to be a *coordinator* of whatever is necessary, such as appointments, medication refills, etc. You may feel overwhelmed, as they rely on you in so many ways, but you are not alone. Enlist help from others such as family, friends, teachers, or anyone else willing to assist. You will be surprised at the help and concern others will offer.

You'll soon learn how widespread this illness called depression is in our society today. Approach the school for help so time lost at school can be kept to a minimum. Look into family leave from your job if you find it necessary to stay home for a period of time. This was a lifesaver for us.

Trust your own judgment and intuition. You know your loved one better than anybody. Follow the doctor's advice, but don't be afraid to disagree or question. Your opinion and ideas are invaluable. (We replaced a sleeping pill that gave Cait nightmares with an herbal remedy; it worked.)

Don't underestimate the power of nurturing to heal the person and shrink the beast. I believe this is just as important as medicine and counseling. Start thinking of yourself as a *nurturer* and experience the good feelings you get in return. Along with doing these loving and caring things goes the gradual "release" toward independence, which is the ultimate goal.

Your battle with the beast of depression won't be an easy one, but you'll find the journey itself has many rewards. We did and so can you!

Best of luck,

Maureen

Maureen Irwin

A Letter from Cait's Brother

Dear Reader,

At the time Cait began going through her depression, I was 16. I didn't really know what was going on. My life was busy with school, work, and sports. It was football season. When I did begin to understand the situation, dealing with it was just too hard to handle.

I was afraid of disrupting my own life. Family counseling was pointless because I wasn't the crazy one and going to see Cait in the hospital was scary. I wondered what my friends were thinking and saying. Sometimes it seemed she had brought it all on herself.

As I look back with some maturity, Cait's situation seems different to me now. If I could go back in time, I would "be there" for her and I would also listen and believe her without judgment. One thing I know for sure is a depressed person needs the whole family to recover.

Andy

Andy Irwin

A Letter from Cait's Dad

Dear Reader,

The easiest thing for a man to do when his child or loved one suffers from depression is to avoid the entire situation. We pretend it doesn't exist and don't want to talk or admit anything is wrong. We feel by avoiding this uncomfortable emotional experience, it will go away. The lyrics to Paul Simon's song pointed out that there are fifty ways to leave your lover. Well, I believe there are just as many ways that men can leave their families and friends suffering from depression.

Why do we act this way? I've suffered myself and done some research on the subject and found that men in general see depression as a weakness. We view it as unmanly and shameful. We're angry with a depressed person because we believe or feel they should be able to "pull themselves out of it." We tend to hide our own depression and seldom seek help and wonder why others should. We usually just live with it and silently suffer, and in some cases, end it all.

The most important thing a person can do is to put the welfare of those struggling with depression ahead of their own fears, anxieties, and preconceived notions about the illness. But I want you to know that it takes real courage to open up and become a team player in the recovery process.

I, personally, didn't have the courage to help Cait through her darkest times. Fortunately, she had others to accept the responsibility and I'll be forever grateful. I couldn't talk about depression then with Cait or anyone else and couldn't be there emotionally for her either. But I did try to help her in my own way.

If your loved one is facing depression, seek ways to help them. If you can't talk about it, don't disappear. If you can't be there emotionally, be there physically and pay attention. Stay in their lives and resist the temptation to avoid their struggle. Don't take your own anger and feelings of helplessness out on them. Build something together, go places, grow things, surf the Net, make plans, make commitments. But most of all, be patient.

Sincerely,

Michael

Michael Irwin

100

A Letter from Cait's Uncle

Dear Reader,

Getting Cait's book into your hands has been a family effort and we hope you've benefited from it in some way. Our family mission is to do everything possible to destigmatize mental illness and help those who suffer from it.

Cait's shameless telling of her own story has become a catalyst for people to open up and talk about either their own personal struggle with depression or about that of a loved one.

Cait's message is simple and real. Mental illness is no different than physical illness. There should be no stigma. Becoming mentally ill can happen to any of us at any time. It's like coming down with pneumonia or, in a milder form, a common cold.

Cait's story has also brought a strong measure of hope to many. And with hope, anything is possible. We also know that her personal victory is not a singular one. With patience, perseverance, and belief in yourself, you can win, too. We wish you well.

All the best,

Uncle Spark

Patrick "Spark" Shaughnessy

Where to Seek Help

American Academy of Child and Adolescent Psychiatry

AACAP is assisting parents and families in understanding developmental, behavioral, emotional, and mental disorders affecting children and adolescents.

202-966-7300

Website: http://www.aacap.org/web/aacp

National Institute of Mental Health (NIMH)

NIMH is dedicated to improving the mental health of Americans; fostering better understanding of effective diagnosis, treatment, and rehabilitation of mental and brain disorders.

301-443-4513

Website: http://www.nimh.nih.gov

National Family Caregivers Association

9621 East Bexhill Drive
Kensington, MD 20895-3104

800-896-3650

Website: http://www.nfcares.org

Institute for Mental Health Initiatives

A nonprofit organization of mental health professionals that promotes emotional well-being in children, families, and their communities.

202-364-7111

Website: http://www.imhi.org

Mood Disorders Support Group, Inc.

MDSG is a nonprofit, self-help organization serving individuals with both depression and manic-depression, as well as their families and friends.

212-533-6374

Website: http://www.mdsg.org

National Foundation for Depressive Illness

The foundation's goals are to educate the public about depressive illness, its consequences and its treatability, and to provide information and referrals to all who make requests.

800-248-4344

Website: http://www.depression.org

National Mental Health Association

NMHA is dedicated to promoting mental health, preventing mental disorders, and achieving victory over mental illnesses through advocacy, education, research, and service.

800-969-6642

Website: http://www.nmha.org

American Association for Marriage and Family Therapy

1100 Seventeenth Street, N.W.
Washington, DC 20016

202-434-2277

The Dana Alliance for Brain Initiatives

The Dana Alliance, a nonprofit organization of more than 185 neuroscientists, was formed to help provide information about the personal and public benefits of brain research.

212-223-4040

Website: http://www.dana.org

Obsessive Compulsive Foundation

P.O. Box 70
Milford, CT 06460

203-874-3843 (24-hour information line)

Website: http://www.iglou.com.fairlight

National Association of Anorexia Nervosa and Associated Disorders (ANAD)

ANAD is the oldest national nonprofit organization helping eating disorder victims and their families. In addition to its free hotline counseling, it operates an international network of support groups for sufferers and families, and offers referrals to health care professionals who treat eating disorders across the U.S. and in fifteen other countries.

847-831-3438

Website:
http://members.aol.com\anad20\index.html

Alcoholics Anonymous World Services

212-870-3400

American Association of Suicidology

American Association of Suicidology is a nonprofit organization dedicated to the understanding and prevention of suicide.

303-692-0985

Website: http://www.suicidology.org

American School Health Association

The mission of the association is to protect and improve the well-being of children and youth by supporting comprehensive school health programs.

216-678-1601

Website: http://www.ashaweb.org

National Institute of Child Health and Human Development

NICHD conducts and supports laboratory, clinical, and epidemiological research on the developmental and behavioral processes that determine and maintain the health of children and adults.

301-496-5133

Website: http://www.nih.gov\nichd

Depression after Delivery

Postpartum depression, education, support, and referrals.

800-944-4773

Website: http://www.msie.yahoo.com

National Alliance for Research on Schizophrenia and Depression

MH interactive asks the Expert, The Write Brain, has chat rooms, mailing lists, and special on-line chat events, as well as continuing education, resources, and the MHI professional directory.

516-829-0091

Website: http://www.mhsource.com

National Organization for Seasonal Affective Disorder

SAD has refined diagnostic criteria and highlighted the heterogeneous nature of the disorder, which causes depression.

303-424-3697

Website:
http://www.mentalhealth.com/book/p40-sad.html

Suicide Prevention Advocacy Network

SPAN is a national grassroots, nonprofit organization bridging all suicide prevention initiatives together to lower suicide rates (especially among young people) in the U.S. and worldwide.

888-649-1366

Website: http://www.spanusa.org

Have a Heart's Depression Resource

Articles on understanding thoughts of suicide, bipolar disorder, mood disorders, and finding help for depression.

Website: http://www.have-a-heart.com

Depression and Related Affective Disorders Association

DRADA's mission is to alleviate the suffering arising from depression and manic-depression by assisting self-help groups, providing education and information, and lending support to research programs.

410-955-4647

Website: http://www.med.jhu.edu.\drada\

Shaky Net Mental Health Resources

SHAKEY is a nonprofit organization dedicated to helping people find the information they need with the greatest possible ease.

Website: http://www.shakey.net

Walkers in Darkness, Inc.

Walkers is a support organization for mood disorders such as major depression and manic-depression. The members range from those who are just starting to come to terms with their illness to those who are long-term sufferers.

Website: http://www.walkers.org

National Depression Screening Project

800-573-4433

To locate free, confidential screening sites near you.

American Foundation of Suicide Prevention

888-333-2377

Suicide prevention research.